REFIRE

Instead of retiring from life,
REFIRE into it.

Six Sure-Fire Ways to Refire
Your Body, Mind & Spirit.

It's Never Too Late to Become More.

By Sharon Morgan Tahaney

Printed in the United States.
First Printing: 2024
ISBN - ISBN Number M0D2077762036

Preface

I feel compelled to preface what you read here by saying -- this is not a book of expert advice coming at you from a source outside yourself. What you will read in these pages is simply the expression of a fellow soul hoping to connect with the knowing that's already inside you. And that *knowing* is this:

it's never too late to become more.

The influencers in my life, no matter from what part of this world they came, have been people of love, of awareness, of gracious giving. While my heart can speak, and your eyes can read – it gives us meaning to share this space right here, right now. It is from the love of you and the love of me that I pass along what I've learned from 50+ role models on how to REFIRE on every level no matter what stage you're in or age you are.

There is a gem here for you. Find it. Feel the love in it. And discover in yourself the spark that will ignite **REFIRED** living so you shine for decades to come.

A bird doesn't sing because it has an answer.

It sings because it has a song.

Chinese Proverb

Acknowledgements

I am a composite of the influence and love of those who have stepped into my life through books, podcasts, live events, or in face to face connections. I'm so grateful for each one of them!

To specifically name a few...I am particularly grateful to the lessons left in my heart by Mary Kay Ash, John Maxwell, Eckhart Tolle, Joe Dispenza, the loving leaders in the Tupperware Corporation, the wise philosophies and love of all the State Queens in the Ms. Senior America organization, my close and loving friends from Texas and Florida, my two bursting-with-passion sons, my sisters who love unconditionally, my best friend who shares wisdom and love so generously, and my parents who taught me to be responsible, patient, and loving. All these influencers have shaped who I am and what I have to share. My voice would be aimless without them.

Content
REFIRE

INTRODUCTION

Have you thought any of this?

> "Why is everyone so angry? So unkind?
> When did it get so hard? It's all too much.
> Just give me my recliner and remote!"

If any of this has passed through your mind, you are like many of us on the wiser side of aging. Given this perspective, you've also likely noticed our counterparts. Some have given up. They feel and act down-right done. Then we see another on the wiser side of aging who are running marathons and walking runways.

What's this about? Why does life (at a certain age) feel full to some and flat to others?

You will get lots of opinions on this one. I'm here to give you six pieces of the puzzle from people who have mapped a pretty good path from business to bliss, corporate to calm, working to waking, and from "I'm old" to "I'm awesome!"

That's the framework for the REFIRE book. One piece of the puzzle for each letter in the word "REFIRE."

These six pieces reveal that living awake, aware and joyful is not a matter of what stage you're in or age you are. It appears from the lessons I'll share here that aging with more life and love than ever before possible is a matter of refiring INTO life rather than retiring *from* it.

I'm reminded of a story I read once of a little girl and her father attending a local fair. They walked by the cotton candy stand and with those little girl eyes sparkling with the desire for the biggest cotton candy made, Dad nodded to the cotton candy maker, and then handed the massive cotton candy to his little girl. As he did, he said, "You may not be able to finish this -- it's as big as you are." Then with the wisdom only a child can share, she said, "Don't worry, Daddy. I'm bigger on the inside than I am on the outside."

Wow, there it is! We have a lot more power than we may imagine. And, maybe, just maybe, that power could mean living well, loving long, and feeling joyful carrying us all the way until the clock runs out on this temporary physical existence. We may be able to finish the whole thing with smiles on our faces. That is, if we recognize that we're bigger on the inside than we are on the outside.

REFIRE is to support that realization. It's an opportunity to grow bigger on the inside and healthier on the outside.

It is time to get refired up in this life of yours, this one right here, right now. I'm sure that's why you're reading this book, which makes me happy! Here's to you and the refiring of your life!

1

Replace "Thinking" With "Knowing" & Turn Off Autopilot

Replacing "thinking" with "knowing" sounds a bit like a riddle. So what does it mean?

I'll give a shot at explaining this most critical and significant aspect of the REFIRE plan. "Thinking" is the language of the brain. The brain, and the product of the brain, this "thinking," belongs to our temporary physical existence. It's a product of our biology. It's provoked by our outside world, and whether negative or positive, it's not reflective of who we really are. It speaks for our ego, the physical side of us.

"Knowing" on the other hand, is the language of the spirit, the part of us that is immortal and made in the image of God. Our bodies are on a clock. Our souls aren't. "Knowing" connects with the timeless part of us that's here forever, the part of our love that's here forever, the purpose of our lives that's here forever. Think about THAT for a minute. What a difference in the power coming from our brain and the power coming from the creative force behind the infinite and collective conscience of the universe.

There's a seismic shift in the power and path revealed to you by choosing to follow your "thinking" vs your "knowing." Here's an example of how this difference plays out in everyday life. Have you ever arrived at your driving destination and realized you didn't remember stopping at the lights or making the turns? Who hasn't, right?

Well, our brains were going full out, chattering up a storm, shifting us into autopilot focused on the past or the future with no chance whatsoever of living in the moment. Allowing our brains to dominate our waking hours is a certain formula for missing the moments, the days, the years, our lives.

So how do you go about replacing thinking with knowing? How do you get off autopilot and shut down the brain long enough, so the spirit has a chance of getting through, of being heard?

Just as a kite will not fly unless it's attached to a string that's grounded by someone holding it, we can't feel, see and live fully aware and present unless we are grounded in the moment. One way I know to be grounded in the moment, is to be still.

Be **still**. Soak up the textures, the colors, the smells, the air, the feeling. Breathe all of it in long and full. Feel the breath and imagine a beautiful shade of pure love, whatever that shade may be for you, being pulled into your lungs from the air in that moment. That's what I do. And when I do, I'm grounded in the present.

Or you could give yourself the gift of meditation. Or take a walk in nature and benefit from the peace of quiet observance. Just still your brain and your thinking for that precious gift of living in the now. I don't know of anyone who shares the power of this gift better than Eckhart Tolle in *The Power of Now*. If you haven't read it, pick up a copy. I'm pretty sure you'll be glad you did.

Being still and getting to the now is where your magnificence lies. It's where your spirit can speak. It's where you can connect with everyone and everything simultaneously and get in contact with the eternal part of you. You'll find peace there and guidance that you may never have thought possible.

I've made a big shift in hearing my spirit by making a big shift in my life. I moved back to the place where I was planted, where I grew up and learned to be human.

I lived in my sweet, little southern home town through high school. Then college and work took me out of state and out of country. I lived decades of doing, getting caught up in the brain chatter and things I wish I'd done and wish I hadn't done or things I needed to do or wanted to do -- focused on the past or the future, and missing the moment. And in a flash, 35 years passed.

Then this very special time we're sharing in our lives introduced me to a new way of thinking – a yearning for peace and simplicity. I was gently drawn into a commitment to myself. The kids had grown up and that burning desire to achieve, to step up to the next rung on the career ladder...was gone. All that felt empty. So ridiculously insignificant. And what was left was a yearning for less – less stuff, less stress, less drama, less chaos -- and a gut-deep desire for peace, love, trust, and harmony. I no longer allowed myself to be with people spewing out negative energy filling the air with toxic anger and criticism. Only those who are committed to contributing rather than criticizing are the ones I choose to influence me.

At this age, I feel how precious moments I've lived really are. I have yearned for those fleeting moments when my sons were young. *Knowing* that is not possible, I'm now dedicated to living *this* moment, off autopilot and fully engaged and present in my life and the love of those surrounding me.

Moving into simplicity turned all that driven *doing* into a quiet calm, a stillness, a *being* never before attainable. My mom had a favorite scripture that's now on her gravestone. "Be still and know that I am God." And here I am *still*, and I *do* know.

In this knowing, I can see the trees on the country road near my parent's home vibrantly green speaking of a force far beyond our own. The birds that sing and the roosters who crow at the same time each morning, all speak of it. The leaves that know just when to fall and the branches that know just when to bud out and renew again in the spring speak of it. The birds that know just when to fly south and return again in the spring speak of it.

The grand plan, the intelligent design becomes so obvious. I don't have to remember to make my heart beat or my food to digest or my hair to grow. There is an intelligence about all of creation that points directly to the creator of the universe. Nothing is by happenstance. The grand plan is a divine plan, and we have the privilege to be a part of it. IF we choose to be...

We can live in it, feel it, and know it, or we can allow our brain chatter to carry us through it unphased and unaware.

I choose to be still. To replace thinking with knowing. And connect to the peace that's beyond all understanding. Join me there and take your first step toward *refiring*.

A Woman Who Lived It

There was a woman who most folks knew as "Aunt Mary Dean." Her name *was* Mary Dean, but she wasn't biologically everyone's aunt. She just felt like a favorite aunt made of pure love which made the title so right.

She seemed to see and hear things the rest of us missed. One night as my family and hers were staying at her Arkansas family home along the

Quachita River, she took my hand and walked outside. The night glistened with stars, the moon burned bright and the lady by my side leaned down and whispered, "Listen to the night. Do you hear it?" And magically, at that moment, I did. I heard the crickets chirp and the branches move in the wind. I saw the moon's glow off the leaves at my feet. I heard my breath move in and out and felt her hand squeeze love around my fingers.

Mary Dean Setliff knew how to live from the spirit and stifle the chatter of her brain – that sassy voice called thinking. I learned at her memorial service that she held the hand of many a child on a night's walk of listening, leading them to the moment of knowing instead of thinking. Aunt Mary Dean died in her 90's leaving behind this first piece of the puzzle in the power of aging with grace and purpose. Let your spirit be the guide. Have faith in your purpose. Trust in the force behind the hum of the crickets, the glow of the moon and the peaceful breath of the moment. Replace "thinking" with "knowing."

2

Easy & Relaxed, Healthy & Positive Will Light Up Your Attitude

Marc Allen wrote a small yet powerful book called, *The Greatest Secret of All*. I read there something that jumped off the page and into my heart. I've put this "greatest secret" into practice each day, and I'm always amazed how it just seems to work.

The practice is to start each day, before you're fully awake while your head is still on your pillow and your brain is open to suggestion, simply say, "Today, in an easy and relaxed, healthy and positive way, I will (fill in the blank with whatever you plan to do that day). Or you could simply say, "Today will be easy and relaxed, healthy and positive."

And guess what. It will be. More accurately, YOU will be. Easy and relaxed, healthy and positive.

Which is exactly why I'm partial to another book called, *Lions Don't Have to Roar.* This book is about projecting a quiet assurance that comes from confidence, competence and real strength. It's about feeling a calmness and grace that will earn you real power, the same kind a lion has. He doesn't have to roar to gain respect. Neither do you.

And here's why feeding your mind with confidence-building information and uplifting concepts can work so powerfully in your favor. Scientific studies are proving that thoughts alone can improve health, fitness, strength, and your brain chemistry. And why is that important? When you change your brain chemistry, physiological outcomes such as more energy, elevated hormone levels, reduced anxiety and improved immune reactions also happen.

Here's how the scientists lay it out for us. If you bombard your cells with peptides from negative thoughts, you are actually programming your cells to receive more of the same negative peptides going forward. At the same time, while you're building up your receptivity to negative thoughts, you're also lowering the number of receptors of positive peptides. The bottom line – you're making yourself more inclined toward negativity.

Here's the good news. Science also provides us some hope. Your cells in your body are replaced on a consistent basis. So, you can reprogram negative hungry cells to be more optimistic by practicing positive thinking. Two powerful positive practices are *living in the moment* and *expressing gratitude*, two REFIRING approaches in your hands right now.

Just in case we have skeptics or simply the curious about the science of Epigenetics, here's a bit more of the science behind this discussion.

The field of Epigenetics shows us that genes are actually switched on or off depending on your experiences. That doesn't say the genes you were born with are altered. It means, however, the hundreds of proteins and other chemicals that regulate your cells ARE changed, regulated upward or downward.

Think about this: Approximately 5 percent of gene mutations are thought to be the direct cause of health issues. The other 95 percent of genes linked to disorders can be influenced depending on life factors. Some of these may be beyond your control, but some are directly in your control, such as exercise, diet, and stress management. The encouraging part of this discussion is this --- your genes alone don't dictate your destiny. Their activity, however, is largely determined by YOU -- your thoughts, attitudes and actions. How great is that! You have a choice in how your genes act based on what you feed them! The more positive the input, the more positive the output of your genes.

That's the reason for this chapter! Epigenetics is proving how powerful your start of each day can be to your physical health and ultimately your personal joy. Choose easy and relaxed, healthy and positive and help your genes to act in your favor.

And one more piece of support to pass along as you change your perspective in order to change your physiology. John Maxwell, the guru of leadership having written scores of books on the topic, suggests you start your day with your "Daily Dozen" to amp up your positive mindset and healthy outcomes. He suggests you create and then read a list of 12 things you're committed to living on a daily basis. He makes your list feel soft and doable by suggesting you start each item with the words, "Just for today, I will…".

Here's my Daily Dozen I wrote 20 years ago and is now on my fridge for easy reference:

1)   I will honor myself by being honest
2)   I will show humanity by being kind to myself and all living things.
3)   I will value differences.
4)   I will thank God for my blessings
5)   I will laugh.
6)   I will try to understand before being understood. (Thanks, Stephen Covey)
7)   I will learn.
8)   I will hear, see, and feel every moment.
9)   I will stand up for my beliefs and respect the beliefs of others.

REFIRE

1.   I will be active.
2.   I will be generous.
3.   When people are their least lovable, I will give them the most love.

Take a minute and write down your Daily Dozen to start your day in an easy and relaxed, healthy and positive way. Put your list so you can see it daily. As you pass by, read it. Then just for today, live it.

The essence of it all is to realize you have the power to shape your day, more accurately, to shape how you *approach and respond* to each day. Take it easy. Make it relaxed. Go for healthy. And always choose positive. When you do, your genes will start acting in your favor and your life will begin to REFIRE on every level.

3

Find Something Hard to Do & Get Your Spark Back

When I was growing up I had a horse I rode to my friend's house several days a week after school. Now my friend lived almost across the street, so the trip was an easy one. When we got there, I would jump down and chat with my friend while my horse grazed on the grass. One day, I decided to ride past my friend's house. What do you think my horse did? He stopped where he was used to stopping. He refused to go one step past what had become a comfortable routine.

I'm reminded of that as we talk about stretching and getting out of our comfort zones. It's easy to get used to just getting by. To settle. To make do. The problem with mediocrity is when you set your eyes on it, you're drawn to it. So if you set your sights on the comfortable spot you've experienced a hundred times before, what's going to happen? You'll stop when you get there. Adequate becomes the end game. Repetition the driving force. Not fun. Not inspiring. Not the place for you.

Your job for REFIRED living is to reach so high you

get dizzy. Start a fire – ignite dreams. And be mindful that it's not about the end game. It's is about the reach itself and the *becoming* in the process.

So try this -- stretch your dream rather than dumbing it down. Find your hard thing and just do it!

- ✓ Maybe for you that would be lifting weights.
- ✓ Signing up for the Senior Olympics.
- ✓ Singing a song at church.
- ✓ Reading a 1000 page book.
- ✓ Talking to a stranger.
- ✓ Entering a Ms. Senior America pageant.
- ✓ Learning a new language.
- ✓ Listening to someone with an opposite point of view.

At 66, my "something hard to do" was entering a Ms. Senior America pageant. At first exposure to the idea, I said, "Oh, thank you for thinking of me, but no, that's something I never thought about doing." Then a few weeks later, I got another call on the subject. My friend who had just experienced this for herself explained that it felt like a women's retreat which sounded like fun to me so I said yes.

Then as I wore a Ms. Arkansas sash and crown, I was exposed to the many views on this topic. I see that puzzled expression asking, "Why would anyone enter a beauty pageant at 66 years old?"

Well, here's my answer now that I've experienced it

so fully in my heart and mind. The crown and sash are symbols, not of beauty, but rather, symbols for saying yes to something scary, of saying yes to something outside the ordinary, of saying yes to stretching and growing. At 66, a crown and a sash simply say, "I've learned something, and this is my platform to share. It.

I met state queens from all over the U.S. who literally lit up the room with their love, wisdom, and commitment to service. Not a crown among them spoke of outward beauty, although there was plenty of that too. The sparkle came from the inside, which has proven to be the most beautiful of all.

So my "hard to do" turned out to be rewarding and revealing. It gave me new friends, new ways to serve, and new ways to grow. So now when someone looks at me with that "why" in their eyes, I smile and secretly wish for them the same kind of shake-up that I had. Pushing beyond ordinary can drop some pretty extraordinary gifts in your lap. These gifts may even sparkle, but for sure, they will nudge you forward.

So find your "something hard to do and do it." You'll be amazed at the new strength you'll discover in yourself. Just one more way to be bigger on the inside than you are on the outside! Try it.

Here's Where It Gets Real

I was so blessed to have met Ms.Texas Senior America 2019, Joyce Brown. She is an incredible woman who has inspired so many with her story of overcoming and becoming. In her own words, here is the transformational "hard to do" story in the life of Joyce Brown.

At 59, I started thinking about retirement and what would be next. I knew I wanted to retire, but I also knew I wanted to do something significant.

At 59, I didn't like where I was. I had gained 30 pounds in my fifties. It seemed I needed chocolate and food as a stress reliever. I didn't know what was next, and I was a little depressed about that.

That's when I had an epiphany. Women I knew over 60, seemed old. I wanted more. I finally decided, you don't have to let them define who you are. You can define 60 for yourself. I have an engineering degree which taught me that everything has a root cause. I looked at myself and knew my root cause for weight gain was eating the wrong things and lack of activity.

My answer was to find an eating program that I liked, and a workout. I said I would not use any more excuses and I wouldn't sabotage myself. I got a Health Certification that taught me about sabotaging moves. For instance, I had been rewarding myself with a snack when I lost a few pounds. I was constantly looking for that satisfaction of food. I realized I couldn't do a cheat day because that one cheat meal would turn into another two months of sliding off my plan.

The next part of my answer was to open a boot camp. I found that when put together, a weight management program and a boot camp worked. I was committed. I would pack my lunch and my snacks every day. I would eat my food instead of grabbing fast food.

When I turned 60 four months later, I had lost 30 pounds. I had gained muscle by working out which gave me confidence. In time, I lost 50 pounds.

Before, I would look at a cookie as a reward. Now I look at it as sabotage. If I want a burger, I plan for it. More thought goes into what I eat. I have done this long enough to know I can cheat and then turn it off. This was not easy. It was hard at first, but I did it anyway. Now eating healthy foods and working out consistently is a way of life.

My platform now is to empower and encourage people to step outside their comfort zones and stretch themselves to live their best lives. We should live our lives with intention and purpose. We were not created to live an average life. We were created to be so much more, but we have to overcome fear to become our best selves.

In other words, by identifying your "hard to do" as Joyce Brown did, you may transform into the person you thought was long gone ages ago.

4

Imagine the Next Chapter & Break the Spell of the Rearview Mirror

There is a Native American saying that sums up the "why" of this chapter so very well. The saying is this, "You can't step into the same river twice."

Why is that? Well, here's my take on the answer. The river is constantly flowing and changing. And just as the river is constantly flowing and changing, so are you. Both sides of the experience have changed. It's impossible to step into the same river the same as you were yesterday. You'll never experience the same river the next time you approach it. The river has changed and so have you.

Just as we never will encounter a new day as we did yesterday. Each new day is a new river. Your next chapter is a new river. Your life and all your surroundings are constantly changing.

What will the river look like as you step into it now? What do you want your next chapter in life to be? How does it look? Who will be in it with you? How will you feel? How will you act? How much energy and passion will you have as you live it? Imagine what your answers are to those questions. Really see them. Believe your vision possible. Snuggle into the feeling it gives you. Wrap your arms around the people there with you. Imagine it as real as if it's already happened.

Here is one thing I know for sure. Rereading the last chapter over and over again won't get you back to living it. You're not the same. Those around you are not the same. The circumstances surrounding you are not the same. Pretending you are and they are, is like wrapping your heart and mind around fog in the wind. You just can't get a firm grip on it.

The sad truth is this. Keeping your eyes fixed on the rearview mirror has a predictable outcome. You'll miss a few sunsets and are sure to run into some brick walls. Another truth I've come to realize is this. If you imagine what you want to lie ahead of you, the life you wish for, the joy you dream about, the love you cherish, the health you long for, you'll magnetically be drawn closer to it.

I also know this. Bend-in-the-road kind of change is uncomfortable. It's actually more than that. It's gut wrenching. It's tough to tackle. Staying steady, on the other hand, sticking with the tried and true, the "proven" methods, on-path and in between the lines, feels safe which makes settling into sameness feel right.

Then it happens. You get used to just getting by.

You go numb and less responsive to life and all it has to offer. Less flexible to new ideas. More committed to defending the status quo. Stuck, static and stale. You sacrifice tomorrow for the "safety" of today. Worn out ways have created ruts so deep, your life rides along without a blip on the screen. You're perfectly ok with the repetition, the recliner and the remote.

It's time to become nimble instead of numb. It's time to bend your ways so you create your next chapter into one that inspires you rather than lulls you to sleep.

How do you do that? How do you become light on your feet? Do you have to change your surroundings, the people around you, your stance on issues?

Not necessarily. The river is about you and your reaction to a changing world. It's like having new eyes, the ones you'd have if you read your Christmas cards again in the middle of July. There's new appreciation, acceptance and love. It's not about changing your life, it's about your life changing you.

Again, how do you do that? How do you change with life so you continue to morph into what's next with passion and love? We'll start building the answer by first looking at the barriers.

Unfortunately, we humans have built-in roadblocks to growing and changing. Behavioral Scientists have studied these roadblocks and have put names on them. They say these tendencies keep us re-reading the old chapter rather than imagining the next one. Here are a couple of these quirks that keep us stuck:

Regret Aversion

We'll start with this one. It seems we have more pain around the possibility of losing than we have joy around the possibility of gaining. We constantly fear regretting our decisions. We fear losing something important. We fear looking silly. Feeling silly. Failing. It's called Risk Aversion.

What do you do about it? When you feel it coming on and hear yourself piling up the excuses about risking a different kind of next chapter, suck the power out of fear by addressing it head on. Get right to it by saying, "So what could happen here? Well, I could learn something new, see something different, and bring that newness and growth into my life just as it is right now." Fear will move on when you look at it head on. The very act lowered your risk aversion and changed you just enough for the new river on your journey.

Status Quo Bias

Being afraid of risk isn't the only hurdle to making your next chapter your best chapter. Another giant roadblock is a Status Quo Bias to keep out the "scary" of something new.

Status Quo Bias simply means we have a tendency to value the way things are over any other choice, even when the "other choice" is clearly preferable. We just like it the way it is. Comfy and familiar. When choice comes down to action, we get stuck in the Status Quo Bias and like things just as they are.

How do you overcome this tendency? You do as the title of this chapter says. You imagine with every bit of color and depth what you want in coming years. You make your next chapter as real as the chair you're sitting in. Own it, feel it, know that it's real, and you'll begin to value it. It will start feeling like it's already yours, and guess what? Your Status Quo Bias starts working in favor of this "imagined" reality. If it feels real, the Status Quo roadblock turns into a force of creation moving you into what's next. That's when you step right into tomorrow's river with ease.

To sum it up, fear is not your friend. Letting go of it will be your greatest ally. For me, my strongest tool in negating the grip of fear is to connect the fear-triggering action to my greater purpose. I take the doing of this scary thing into how the doing of it could benefit someone else. Eleanor Roosevelt once said that if you think about your purpose and how it can help someone else, you'll forget about the fact your knees are knocking. Her knees were probably knocking when she found herself married to the President of the United States and chairing the UN Commission on Human Rights. But she did it anyway. Her "next chapter" was one in which she soared, fear or no fear.

That brings me to an eye-opening study that proves the powerful role mindset has on aging. The study has been called "The Counter Clockwise Study" and was conducted by Ellen J. Langer and a group of Harvard students. It's outlined in her book, *Mindfulness*, a must-read for anyone interested in the science of "being bigger on the inside" and the impact it has on aging.

Here's the essence of this study. The question to be answered was this, "Could physiological factors associated with aging, be improved by psychological factors? Are aging processes less fixed than we may have thought?

To answer this question, two groups of men aged 75 were chosen to participate in a weeklong study. In this week, these men were placed into two groups, the Experimental group and a Comparison group.

The Experimental group, was completely immersed in 1959, and were asked to live in 1959 as they were 25 years younger. They were taken to a country retreat, shown movies from 1959, magazines surrounded them from that year, political speeches from 1959 were discussed, photographs of all participants were shared as they appeared 25 years younger. The key here is that they could only speak in present tense about 1959. They could not discuss anything past that year and lived for that week in their imagined 1959.

The Comparison group were surrounded by 1959 elements also, but this group was able to talk in past tense about these experiences. They looked back but were also able to look forward and talk about themselves and events happening after 1959.

What were the results of this immersion into 1959, with one group completely involved with 1959 as a present tense experience truly living and believing they were indeed 25 years younger? And how did their results compare to the comparison group who looked back in a past tense sort of way through eyes that were 25 years older? Can an imagined state alter physiological aging? Can the state of a person's body be turned back if we shift that person's mindset to 25 years younger?

The Experimental group, who lived and talked as if they were 25 years younger, had these results over the Comparison group who looked back at 1959 as a memory rather than as an imagined state of being. For the Experimental group:
- Hearing improved
- Hand strength increased
- Finger length increased in a third of the group and remained the same in the remainder of the group while a third of the Comparison group actually worsened on this

measurement
- The Experimental group had a greater increase in seating height
- Greater mental dexterity
- And improvements on intelligence tests

Ellen Langer seems to have shown in this "Counter Clockwise" Study that the so-called irreversible signs of aging can be altered through psychological factors. Assumptions of how someone grows old may be exactly why we experience these assumed "irreversible" signs of aging.

If we didn't feel compelled to carry out these limiting perceptions of aging, we just might have a better shot of replacing years of decline with years of growth and purpose. In other words, we would replace retiring from life into REFIRING into it!

5

Reset Your Internal Thermostat BEFORE You React

Here's a simple fact we've all come to realize. People say and do dumb stuff. Well, we think it's dumb because we don't like or agree with it. They think it's brilliant and perfect. Therefore, arguing the point is useless. Instead, what do you do when people say or do (you know) dumb stuff?

We can't control it. We can't even change their minds about it. The only thing we CAN do is control how we react to it.

That's it. That's what you control. Period. So, let's pick up and examine what's in our control, our reaction.

Let's just say, someone is coming at you hot. They are passionate and merging on angry. Their opinion is a 180 from your own (you know, the dumb stuff), and you are standing there on the receiving end. Good news! You have a way to turn the temperature of the conversation to chill or to warm!

Remember, you're not trying to change their minds or what comes out of their mouths, just how you feel about it. Think of yourself as having this internal thermostat. It's got one of those locked plastic boxes over it and only you have the key. Now, they're coming at you hot, so you simply reach for your internal thermostat (it magically unlocks when you "reach" for it). And you turn your internal thermostat to CHILL.

That's better. You can even give yourself a moment to actually feel the chill by saying something like, "Well, that's an interesting perspective. Give me a moment to process that." Continue in a "chill" setting and watch the temp cool off in the room. The person with the "dumb" perspective will start feeling a cooling effect and even though there is no mind shift, there is a climate shift. You're chill, and you can choose to move forward and have a productive conversation. Or not. Either way, you are calm, cool and fully in charge of your attitude.

Or let's say someone you meet is as cold as ice. They have a barrier up and you know meeting them with that same icy reception is simply going to freeze out any hope of connection. Remember your internal thermostat again and turn it to WARM. Be warm, ask loving questions, maybe extend a loving hand. Here's a simple truth. People who are at their least lovable, need the most love. So, send out love, and watch how you warm a room and possibly even a relationship.

REFIRE

I'm reminded of the movie, The Horse Whisperer. Robert Redford's character had a way with wild horses or highly disturbed horses by simply controlling his own internal thermostat. Remember the scene when the highly disturbed horse ran wildly away from him in the pasture. Redford took a seat on the ground with his back turned humbly to the horse. Over time, the horse sensed the warmth and humility floating in the air from Redford's posture and attitude. With gentle movement and loving intentions, Redford found himself with the horse's nose nuzzling his left ear. When people (or horses) are at their least lovable, that's when they need the most love. Walk gently, drop all force, speak with love letting go of the outcome and only controlling your own internal thermostat, and watch relationships bloom.

Beyond your attitude, there may be need for actual words to talk your way through a tough conversation. Here's one that's worked for me.

When I was faced with a crucial conversation with my boss once, I prepared by picking up a book appropriately named, *Crucial Conversations, Tools for Talking When the Stakes Are High* by Kerry Patterson. Great read.

I came away with an acronym that has served me well on many occasions. That acronym for guiding a crucial conversation according to Patterson, is STATE.

REFIRE

S reminds us to begin by Stating the facts as you see them. (eg. *I see you didn't get to the meeting yesterday or make the call we'd set up this morning.*)

T reminds us to Tell your impression. (eg. *I'm getting the feeling that your goals or interests are shifting a bit.*)

A reminds us to Ask if you have it right. (eg. *Am I on target with that?*)

T reminds us to Talk tentatively. Patterson so eloquently says, "You can be abrasive or persuasive, but not both at the same time." So put your guns in your holster and speak gently. (eg. *I may be off or not reading this right. Is there anything to what I'm saying here?*)

E reminds us to Extend an invitation for a win. Simply end your part on a note that's open for more. (eg. *How about we pull together again and set up our next (whatever) next Tuesday at 11. Does that work for you?*)

REFIRE

- S
  State the facts as you see them
- T
  Tell your impression
- A
  Ask if you have it right
- T
  Talk Tentatively
- E
  Extend invitation for a win

I like this tool for moving over hazardous ground in relationships. Remember, keep your internal thermostat top of mind, control it according to the situation, and if you have to use words to get through a tough conversation, think of STATE. Your relationships will love you for it!

6

Express Gratitude & Get Your Joy Back

Here's a big one – the most transformative REFIRE I've ever experienced. This REFIRE lesson is about adapting from grief to gratitude.

I'll start by turning to the dragonfly. It adapts. It's the only living thing that survives in all three dimensions of our environment. Born underwater, it then climbs to the surface to dry its wings. And, when its wings are ready, it takes to the sky.

REFIRE

My REFIRE of adapting began when my son's wings were ready. It was a rainy Sunday afternoon in Orlando, Florida and my son, 24, was driving his car around a sharp curve. His car skidded off the road and into a Cypress tree.

His physical life ended there at that Cypress tree. His wings were ready.

Too, too soon. How could those wings be ready when I was so utterly not? It was so very heavy. I didn't know how to stand up under it.

Before I share the rest of this journey, I'd like to share why I'm addressing it at all in this REFIRE book.

I've discovered that there are many just like me who are forced to make this journey, ready or not. A recent study conducted by the Chicago-based group called The Compassionate Friends categorized all child deaths from miscarriage through the death of an adult child. It found that 19 percent of adults have experienced the death of a child. That 19% would be about 46 million people who have lost a child. Too many who may find some comfort here. That's why I'm sharing this story.

So here goes, just as my spirit dictated it. My brain wanted to edit and organize it in a more logical way. But logic just doesn't fit this discussion, so here is my journey just as it played out...

Losing a child is like losing yourself. The person you were is gone forever. You move through stages to get to that truth. You start where you think you can't possibly live. The pain is too great to survive. Then you pass through the stage of functioning, making the motions, existing. During this time, you may experience a spark of joy. My grandson hugged me and I felt it. It actually surprised me, but I realized I could feel joy. This new person I was could feel joy!

And the truth of that moment is this. The new person you are is entirely different and must live entirely differently. The old life is gone. Now it's up to you to make this new person, the one forged out of red-hot pain, the one you've built out of ashes, to be better than the you before. That's a big mission. How do you get here? How do you find yourself?

How do you struggle through the pain, the shock, the realization, the gut-wrenching movement from that moment of loss to the rest of life? I'm sharing it in hopes it helps in the healing of others on this path.

If you've lost someone, actually lost them from this earth, to a place where you can't text, call or visit them. You can't rub a shoulder or kiss a cheek or get caught in the gleam of a look. All of it is gone. The person is gone. You think they're coming back for a long, long time. You feel that they are coming back. They must come back.

But they don't. What was left for me was a vacuum. A hole. An after-draft that sucked in my spirit. I got caught in the current of the passage. And in that vacuum, in that pulling along, in that middle place, that after-draft, I was changed. That thin veil between the earthly and the spiritual was ripped open, and in that gap, I saw new things, felt new depth, sensed the spirit that was still alive even without the bodily coat that wrapped it once upon a time. I got an up-close and extremely personal hand in hand relationship with God. And the very fabric of my being morphed with the movement.

If you've lost someone like that, you already know what I mean. That ache that cut through the curtain where the light is, where spirits catch the wind and finger-paint the clouds in the sky, where freedom dances with no constraints. That place. It had some meaning for us before the light shone through from the after-draft, but now it's real. It's right here with us. We feel it and see it. God grants us that -- these gifts of seeing the one we loved so purely on earth whispering a little bit of truth from their new home.

When a love left, part of you left with it. The carbon composition remained, but your spirit got caught in the passage.

You may know this. You may be living this right now. I'm so sorry.

If you haven't lived this, I'm so grateful for that. However, I want you to know what those caught in

33

the after-draft know. When you do, the things you
see, the people you have, the days you spend can
be lifted above the now. That now seems reality
forever, that deep in-the-gut satisfaction you're not
even aware you have, becomes even more
precious and the learnings that were seared into me
are gifted to you as well.

Here are a few of them. It's not about what we do,
how much we make, the stuff we accumulate.
When we come to the moment we're ripped clean of
all of it, what will be left is what matters – our true
essence, our unadorned soul.

And it's that soul, the spirit that becomes free of the
body, it's that move out of body and into the wind of
the world that creates the light of the after-draft.
And it's the light our after-draft creates that is the
very purpose of the life we now live.

Maybe, standing in this light, we will no longer settle
for existing, getting by, scrambling through lists,
leaning into the wind, focusing on finish lines.
Maybe, we will become shockingly awake,
awesome, and begin to live like it.

Now this brings me to the most transformative
REFIRE of my life. This stage of my journey meant
turning grief for the loss into soft soothing gratitude
for the life.

How did this adaptation happen? From being
completely underwater and numb, to living earthly

again among people and jobs and friends, and then finally turning my eyes upward to see this most unimaginable painful tragedy from God's perspective? And finally allowing the spiritual to overtake the earthly. And gratitude to overtake grief. How does this progression happen?

A friend of mine who had lost her son some 15 years earlier shared this great wisdom. "If you can turn the grief for the loss into gratitude for the life, you will live again and smile again and maybe even laugh again."

So, I took her words to heart and into practice. I prayed day after day, "Thank you, God, for the 24 years I did have with my son. Thank you for his twinkly brown eyes, his crazy antics, his hard lessons and his soft lessons. Thank you for the "I love you, Mom" he said at the end of every phone call. I thanked God for every aspect of my son.

And as that shift from grief to gratitude happened, so did my life begin again. I could talk about him without crying. I could even laugh when remembering his humor and unorthodox antics.

It was as if I was that little rock given me by my son when he was five as we walked together on a gravel road near our home. He reached down and immediately handed it to me saying, "This one's for you." That rock had been shaped into a perfect heart as if by an artist with great precision and intention. That rock among all the others on that gravel road had experienced friction. It had its edges knocked off and ground down by the sand, rain and other rocks. And all that was left was this perfect heart.

Just as with all of us. The friction of illness, or loss, or relationships gone wrong – whatever the cause, the friction of our living chips off the rough edges and all that's left – if we're paying attention – is the essence of our being, the heart of the matter, our eternal soul.

And that's the REFIRE that transforms us into why we're here. To learn and grow and become, until finally, we are shaped into the perfect heart.

Here are the stages again, and my wish for you if you've been forced to take this journey, is that you've traveled through the first two stages and are finding yourself moving to relief, wakefulness and gratitude. Here, again, are the stage:

1. It's just too heavy
2. We adapt to the weight and just exist,
3. We find some **relief** from the vacuum of absence
4. We become **awake** to the spiritual, and
5. **Grateful** for the gift of life.

7

To Sum It Up…Get a Bit WILD in the Days to Come

To wrap up the big thoughts of this book about REFIRING, think of getting a bit WILD in the days to come.   WILD is used as an acronym here, so it means something different than what may have come to your mind just now.

"One of my favorite books growing up was *Call of the Wild* by Jack London. It was all about relationships, loyalty, grit, leadership, love, and animals. I value all those and have found them to be important in my life. I've owned dogs my entire life, grew up with a horse, and adopted another horse for a therapeutic riding center. This "call of the wild" has merged with my career urging me to share lessons I consider to be the best I could pass along to others.

I believe leaders, successful leaders, will always

have a wild side. They will never be trapped by self-imposed limitations. They will always break out of scarcity cages and into the freedom of abundance. They will open up to what's around the corner, let go of their fears, laugh loudly and often, and embrace themselves to be fully who they are. They will be wild.

So I would like to leave you with a lesson from the "call of the wild." It starts with being full of...

Wonder

Inspiring,

Loud in your vision and

Delicious in your spirit

Let's break all this down...

Wonder-Full
Being full of wonder is a precious gift to give yourself. You see things you would never see if you let yourself fall into the jaded, rolling-eyes response, or get trapped longing for the past or wishing for the future. Being full of wonder means seeing things as if they're brand new, as if it's your first time, amazed by the power of the moment. It's the difference between flying through holiday cards in the midst of shopping, wrapping, decorating, cooking and doing all the normal thousand things in the month of December. It's the difference between all that, and taking your holiday cards out on the beach the following July. You'll likely see so much more than

you did in December. Being full of wonder is about being in the moment with a focused attention on the now. Living in the present being open and fully aware. There is nothing more precious than now when you're living full of wonder. It will make every experience powerful and every person the *only* person.

Inspiring

You've probably picked up this next point in this book by now. I'm a real believer that motivation, not legislation, will move people forward. Rules will never be the reason someone follows you. What will be the reason is how closely you connect with their inner most desires, concerns, dreams, and hopes. Connecting is not about power. It's about empowerment, which simply means connecting with the dreams of others and the inner strength they have in fulfilling those dreams. That's when you inspire. When you get inside, beneath the fear, and discover greatness. The word "inspire" originally meant, "breathe." That's what you do when you inspire. You breathe life into dreams.

Loud in your vision

A leader's voice must be heard above the noise of the everyday. Leaders carry the vision, the belief and the path. Speak it out. Be obvious about your goals and desires. Share them with your family, friends, and colleagues. You must shine so others find their way through you. One of my favorite songs as a child was "This little light of mine, I'm going to let it shine." It reminds me we must let our lights shine. Not for the purpose of stepping into the spotlight, but for the purpose of shining the light on someone else. Be loud in your vision so you light the way for others.

Delicious in your spirit

And finally, a leader must be delicious in spirit. You must attract people to you for what they can gain from being around you. You're like honey. No one can resist because of the sweet gifts they receive when they're with you. This is the law of the harvest. When you give, you receive. So, give without expecting anything in return. That's when you will attract people to come into your life. That's when you'll enjoy the delicious rewards of a delicious spirit.

⑧

Epilogue

The Ultimate REFIRE Secret

There was a horse originally named Midnight who came from a bloodline having three Triple Crown winners. He should have been magnificent on the racetrack. But he wasn't. As a result, his owners saw no value in him and left him to literally fade away and die.

But instead of losing his life, he actually found it. A therapeutic riding facility in Shreveport, Louisiana rescued him. And his real story began. The story of Midnight and a little girl who, because of one another, each discovered greatness.

The little girl was born with a chromosomal disorder and her parents were told she would never speak or walk. Then when she was five, the family discovered therapeutic riding. Overcoming fear and physical struggle, this little girl got on the back of a horse. Then it happened. She spoke. And the first word she spoke was the name of the horse she was riding. She's been riding ever since. And now she rides the horse with the Triple Crown bloodline and failed racing career.

41

She has given him value again. And he has given her strength. His story now matters not because he stood in the Winner's Circle, but because he walks for a higher purpose. And not because of his regained strength, but because of the strength he's released in the little girl on his back.

Which points to the ultimate REFIRE secret. It comes from both giving and getting. From spirit and strength. From heart and mind. There's a duality to it. This long game of aging and short game of living.

Trust in your long game. But live in the short game – this moment. And you're sure to find the ultimate REFIRE secret. **The longer your view and shorter your focus, the greater the gifts you'll have for others.**

In short...
LIVE ALL OUT so you can GIVE OUT ALL!

21 Sure-REFIRE Moves

1. Be aware, awake and present in each moment. That's this one. This one right now.
2. Know your purpose – your greatest gift you came here with as a human being.
3. Now give that gift away. The more you give in life, the more you get from life.
4. Keep in mind that a conversation is NOT about you.

5. Love your neighbor as yourself. You've heard that plenty, but really do it. And do it by loving yourself, so you CAN love your neighbor.
6. Get ahead by putting other people first.
7. Build trust by being trustworthy.
8. Stretch your goals and dreams rather than dumbing them down.
9. Never let the magic of the moment slip into ho-hum. This moment. Right now. (I know I said this already, but the thought is worth repeating)
10. Be human -- the kind you would like to share a tent with.
11. Start doing your next thing before you're ready. Just start. You can edit, tweak, and adjust later. Just start.
12. You get what you work for. Wishes don't work unless you do. So, work for what you want.
13. Stop whining. It doesn't change a thing except the annoyance level of everyone in ear shot.
14. Don't depend on stuff to make you happy. Stuff fills your surroundings, not your heart.
15. Read good books. Get in there with the deep thinkers.
16. Understand in a bone-deep, gut-level way that what you send into the lives of others, WILL come back into your own. Simple karma, baby.
17. Imagine that each person you meet has four words in neon lights running across his/her

forehead. Those four words: "Make Me Feel Important." (thanks, Mary Kay Ash)

18. When things go wrong (and they will), instead of saying, "This sucks!" say, "Wow, here's a new lesson I get to learn."

19. The best answer to a good conversation is always a question. Ask a question and LISTEN. Then ask another one, and LISTEN.

20. Believe people are good and their intentions are good too. Polyanna it! Scrooging it isn't nearly as much fun!

21. All the darkness in the world can not extinguish a single candle. Be sure your candle remains shining. The world needs it!

REFIRE is for seniors at or near retirement who wonder if life is about to be full or flat. REFIRE outlines six pieces of the puzzle from people who have mapped a pretty good path from working to waking and from "I'm old" to "I'm awesome!" You'll find here one piece of the puzzle for each letter in the word, "REFIRE." No matter what stage you're in or age you are, REFIRE will reveal how to refire *INTO* life rather than retiring *from* it.

Made in the USA
Middletown, DE
09 September 2024